KT-463-275

Department of Health
Scottish Office Home and Health Department
Welsh Office

Drug Misuse and Dependence

Guidelines on Clinical Management

Report of a Medical Working Group

London: HMSO

© Crown copyright 1991

First published 1991

ISBN 0 11 321376 X

"a change in professional . . . attitudes to drug misuse is necessary as attitudes and policies which lead to drug misusers remaining hidden will impair the effectiveness of measures to combat the spread of HIV"

(Advisory Council on the Misuse of Drugs 1988).

"it is . . . unethical for a doctor to withhold treatment from any patient on the basis of a moral judgement that the patient's activities or lifestyle might have contributed to the condition for which treatment was being sought. Unethical behaviour of this kind may raise the question of serious professional misconduct"

(General Medical Council statement on "HIV infection and AIDS: the ethical considerations." paragraph 7. August 1988).

Potential Medical Contacts of a Drug Misuser

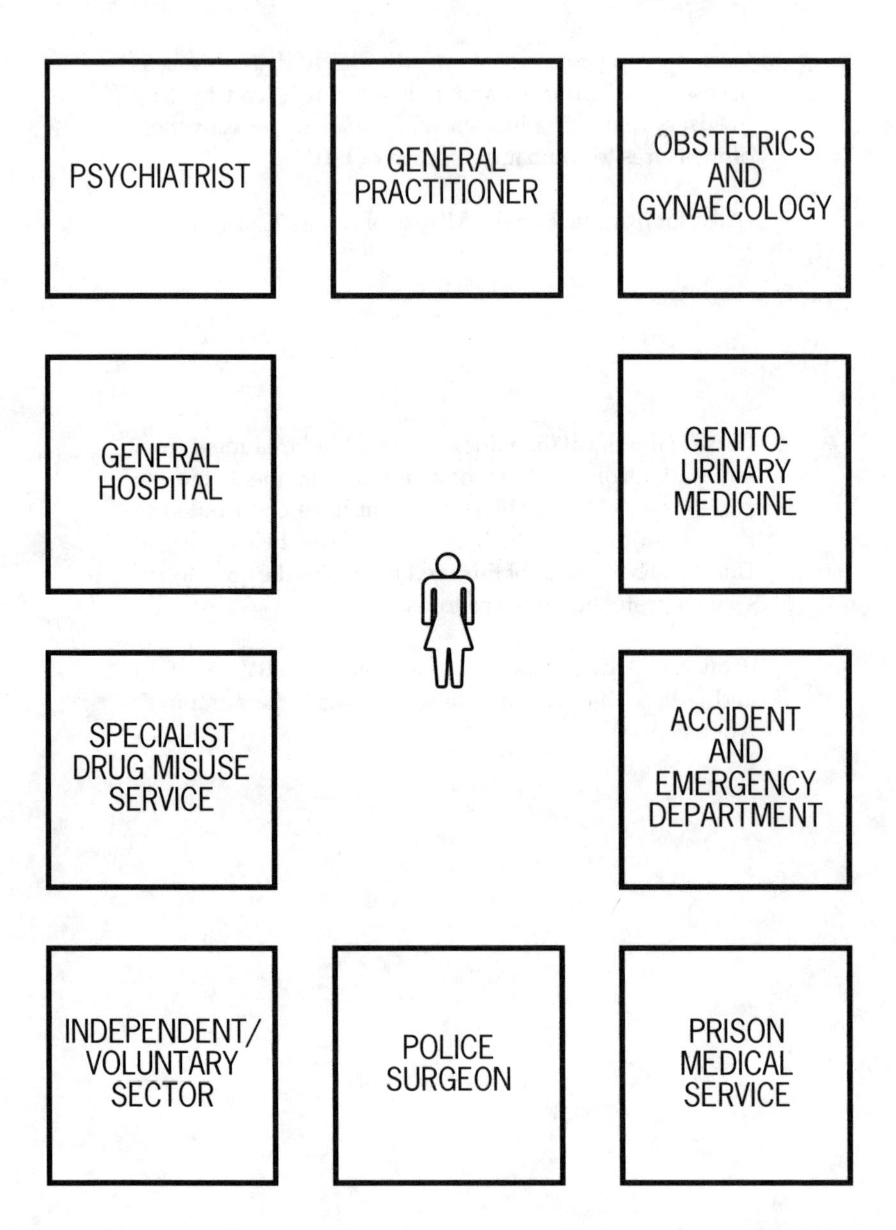

CONTENTS

MEDICAL WORKING GROUP

Chairman

Dr. John Strang
Consultant Psychiatrist, Bethlem Royal and Maudsley Hospital, London; and Consultant Adviser to the Chief Medical Officer on Drug Misuse.

Members

Dr. David Curson
Consultant Psychiatrist, Royal Masonic Hospital, London.

Professor Charles George
Professor of Clinical Pharmacology, University of Southampton.

Professor Hamid Ghodse
Professor of the Psychiatry of Addictive Behaviour, St. George's Hospital Medical School, London.

Professor David Grahame-Smith
Rhodes Professor of Clinical Pharmacology, University of Oxford; and Chairman of the Advisory Council on the Misuse of Drugs.

Dr. Judy Greenwood
Consultant Psychiatrist, Royal Edinburgh Hospital, Edinburgh.

Dr. David Hawkins
Consultant Physician (Genito-urinary Medicine), St Stephen's Clinic and Westminster Hospital, London.

Dr. Roy Robertson
General Practitioner, Muirhouse Medical Group, Edinburgh.

Dr. Mary Rowlands
Senior Medical Officer, HM Prison, Bristol.

Dr. Vipin Trivedi
General Practitioner, Devi Surgery, Southport.

Professor Peter Tyrer
Professor of Community Psychiatry, Mental Health Unit, St Charles Hospital, London.

Observers

Mr. Alan MacFarlane
Chief Inspector, Drugs Inspectorate, Home Office.

Dr. John Basson
Principal Medical Officer, Scottish Office Home and Health Department.

Secretariat

Dr. John Shanks
Principal Medical Officer, Department of Health.

Dr. Robyn Young
Senior Medical Officer, Department of Health.

Mr. Michael O'Connor
Higher Executive Officer (Development), Department of Health.

Acknowledgements

The Working Group is grateful to the many individuals and organisations who provided expert advice during the production of these Guidelines.

Summary

1 Introduction

1.1 The task of the Medical Working Group was to revise the Guidelines of Good Clinical Practice in the Treatment of Drug Misuse in the light of developments since its publication in 1984.

1.2 The Guidelines are written by doctors for doctors in general. They offer suggestions which doctors can interpret in the context of their own clinical practice.

1.3 The Guidelines cover misuse of, or dependence on, Controlled Drugs, prescribed drugs and legally-available substances.

2 Drug Misuse and Dependence

2.1 Drug misuse is a substantial and growing problem.

2.2 Patterns of drug misuse have changed since 1984. Opioids remain a growing problem. More recent drugs of misuse include Ecstasy, crack, buprenorphine and benzodiazepines.

2.3 Drug misusers are a heterogeneous group of people. They include adolescents experimenting with drugs, illicit drug users whose lives are centred on drugs, stable long-term drug users and patients who have become dependent on prescribed drugs.

2.4 Doctors have a role in the primary prevention of drug misuse and in its clinical management. Straightforward aspects of clinical management can be taken on by any doctor; more complicated interventions are best tackled by doctors with the relevant additional training.

3 Principles of Clinical Management (for all doctors)

These principles apply to all forms of drug misuse and dependence.

3.1 Every doctor is now likely to see patients who misuse drugs. Effective intervention encourages recovery and reduces the risk of HIV infection and other harm. (Table 3.1)

3.2 Every doctor should address the general health needs of his patients who misuse drugs, including straightforward treatments for drug dependence such as methadone withdrawal from opioids. Clinical management aims to help the patient deal with drug-related problems, reduce the risks from continuing drug use and support the patient towards becoming drug free. (Table 3.2)

3.3 At the first interview, a patient may not declare a problem of drug misuse. The doctor should be prepared to enquire about drug misuse and should be alert for features which suggest it. (Table 3.3) A careful history and physical examination is essential. Advice should be offered on harm minimisation (3.5.1) and any necessary immediate treatment given.

3.4 Doctors are obliged by law to notify the Addicts Index of contact with opioid and cocaine addicts and should also report details of patients with any recent drug problem to the Regional Drug Misuse Database.

3.5 HIV makes it especially important to attract more drug misusers into treatment. "Harm minimisation" aims to reduce the damage from drug misuse. (3.5.1 Tables 3.4 and 3.5) The doctor should take appropriate precautions to prevent transmission of blood-borne viruses such as HIV and Hepatitis B during health care procedures. (3.5.2) Prescribing a substitute drug can be an effective intervention but should always form part of a broader strategy of care. Prescribing may follow a pattern of rapid withdrawal, gradual withdrawal or maintenance. (3.5.3) The doctor should review the available options where a patient fails to improve. (3.5.4)

3.6 Doctors who may see patients who have overdosed must have ready access to opioid antagonists. Compulsory admission to hospital under the Mental Health Act may be justified for a drug misuser who is also suffering from mental disorder. Drug misuse alone is not sufficient grounds.

3.7 The doctor should ask for advice from, or referral to, a specialist in drug misuse where the patient's condition or care are more complicated. (Table 3.6)

3.8 Services should be arranged to avoid congregation of large numbers of drug misusers.

4 Special Circumstances

4.1 *Primary Care:* There is a balance to be struck between making help readily available to those in urgent need while maintaining appropriate vigilance to avoid abuse of the service. Shared care with a specialist in drug misuse is often appropriate.

4.2 *Accident and Emergency Care:* The A&E Department should have a policy on responding to requests for drugs or injecting equipment. Patients who have overdosed (see 3.6) or who require sedation should be admitted. Where possible, advice should be obtained from the local drug misuse service and the patient's GP informed.

4.3 *General Hospital Care:* A patient admitted to general hospital may be reluctant to volunteer a history of drug misuse. The emergence of unrecognized withdrawal symptoms can cause diagnostic difficulties. Prescribing too large a dose of substitute drugs increases dependence while too little may encourage self-medication or premature self-discharge. There should be an early assessment of the need for advice from the local drug misuse service.

4.4 *Pregnancy and Neonatal Care:* Antenatal care should be planned to take account of the opportunities and risks. (4.4.1.) Skilled paediatric care should be available during and after delivery (4.4.2 and 4.4.3.) Breast feeding needs careful consideration in the light of HIV status and drug use. A meeting should be held to plan appropriate support of mother and child. (4.4.4.)

4.5 *General Psychiatric Care:* Drug misuse may be the presenting problem or exist as co-pathology with mental illness. There should be clear operational policies on admission, discharge and continuing care.

4.6 *Genito-urinary Medicine and HIV services:* Good liaison between doctors in HIV services and doctors in drug misuse services is essential to ensure adequate care for drug misusers living with HIV.

4.7 *The Independent Sector:* Doctors should seek peer support from senior colleagues and ensure consistent standards and adequate access to consultation with local NHS services. Doctors need to be aware of the potential pitfalls of receiving payment for treatment of drug misuse. Patients should live within easy reach. If prescribing controlled drugs, this is best limited to oral methadone and dihydrocodeine.

4.8 *Police Custody:* Police surgeons will need to provide treatment to prevent or reduce withdrawal symptoms and should inform police officers on the effects and risks of drug use by patients in custody.

4.9 *Prison:* Appropriate detoxification will be required for prisoners who are dependent on drugs. (4.9.1) The prison doctor should provide assessment, information and liaision with community services. (4.9.2)

Appendix 1: *Managing Withdrawal*
Psychological support is important (A1.1.1).
Withdrawal from **opioids** may be possible through the use of less addictive medication (A1.2.1).
If prescription of substitute drugs such as methadone is required, an initial daily dose should be established (A1.2.2) before beginning on a withdrawal schedule.
Withdrawal from **sedative/hypnotic** drugs may be carried out by reduction from an established initial daily dose (A1.3.1).
Diazepam is often a convenient drug to use (A1.3.2).
Additional medication may sometimes be required (A1.3.4).
Withdrawal from **stimulants** is best done by abrupt discontinuation. Insomnia and depression may require treatment (A1.4).
Hallucinogens should be discontinued abruptly. Subsequent psychological disturbance may require treatment (A1.5).

Volatile substances should be discontinued abruptly. (Volatile substance misuse carries a risk of sudden death (A1.6)).
Alcohol is commonly misused together with drugs. Withdrawal is managed as with sedative/hypnotic drugs (A1.7).

Appendix 2: *Notification, Reporting and Prescribing*
Doctors must notify the Addicts Index of any contact with a patient who is addicted to the specified opioids or cocaine.The Index can provide information to the doctor on patients previously notified (A2.1).
The Regional Drug Misuse Databases rely on voluntary reporting; they cover the whole range of drugs of misuse (A2.2).
There are specific regulations for the prescribing of controlled drugs. Special prescription forms allow dispensing by instalments from a single prescription. Any doctor may prescribe methadone and most other controlled drugs to a drug misuser; it is only for cocaine, diamorphine and dipipanone that a special licence is required (A2.3).

Abstract

Sections 1 and 2 set the context and describe the problem.

Section 3 sets out the basic principles of clinical management – these apply to all doctors.

Section 4 specifies how the basic principles of Section 3 relate to particular areas of medical practice.

1 Introduction

1.1 The Medical Working Group

The Medical Working Group was set up in March 1991 by the Department of Health to revise the document "Guidelines of Good Clinical Practice in the Treatment of Drug Misuse" which was published in 1984. Much of the material from the 1984 Guidelines remains relevant and has been incorporated into the present document, but developments such as the emergence of HIV infection among drug misusers required changes to reflect current practice.

Dr John Strang was invited by the Chief Medical Officer to be chairman of the Group. The membership of the Group was drawn from nominations, invited by the Department of Health from representative medical bodies and individuals with appropriate expertise. The Group held four one-day meetings between May and August 1991 and received written evidence from a range of medical and non-medical bodies.

Terms of Reference

To revise the "Guidelines of Good Clinical Practice in the Treatment of Drug Misuse" in the light of developments since 1984, particularly:

(i) the spread of HIV infection among injecting drug misusers;

(ii) the emergence of new patterns of drug misuse;

(iii) new developments in treatment, rehabilitation and prevention.

1.2 The New Guidelines.

1.2.1 Who are they for?

The Guidelines are written by doctors for doctors, and for doctors in general rather than for specialists in drug misuse. The intention is to offer flexible guidance to help all doctors, within the context of their own clinical practice, to provide an effective response to patients with problems of drug misuse. Doctors who specialise in drug misuse should be aware that medical colleagues dealing with drug misusers will require ready access to their advice and assistance. Some doctors might not have access to the full range of support services.

1.2.2 Scope of the Guidelines

The Guidelines cover the misuse of:

- drugs such as heroin, cocaine and LSD which are controlled under the Misuse of Drugs Act 1971.
- legally-available substances such as solvents and butane gas (but not tobacco).
- drugs, such as benzodiazepines, which may have been legitimately prescribed for therapeutic purposes.

Many people with a drug problem also misuse alcohol and vice versa. Guidance for doctors on dealing with alcohol problems is contained in a number of recent publications.[1,2,3]

1.2.3 Terminology

Suggestions, not Instructions.

The style of the Guidelines is sometimes terse in order to be brief and clear. In places they describe statutory obligations which doctors must fulfil. Most of the content is suggestions offered to doctors by a group of medical colleagues for interpretation in the light of the doctors' own situations. The Guidelines are neither a set of rules nor a textbook: doctors will also need access to more detailed information and to specialist advice.

"Drug misuse": is used here to denote drug taking which is hazardous or harmful and unsanctioned by professional or cultural standards. It is broadly equivalent to terms such as "drug abuse" and "problem drug taking"[4].

"Drug dependence": is used more specifically to describe the altered physical and psychological state which results in disturbed physical and mental functioning when the drug is abruptly discontinued. It is broadly equivalent to "addiction". Not all drug misusers are drug dependent.

Drug misusers, like doctors, come in both sexes. The masculine pronoun is used throughout to mean both "him" and "her".

2 Drug Misuse and Dependence

2.1 The scale of the problem

The numbers of addicts notified to the Home Office represent perhaps only 20% of opioid and cocaine users and does not include people who misuse other drugs such as benzodiazepines. Injecting drug misuse is currently the most rapidly-increasing exposure category among people with AIDS. Over 1000 people died in 1989 as a result of drug misuse, drug dependence and poisoning with controlled drugs.[5]

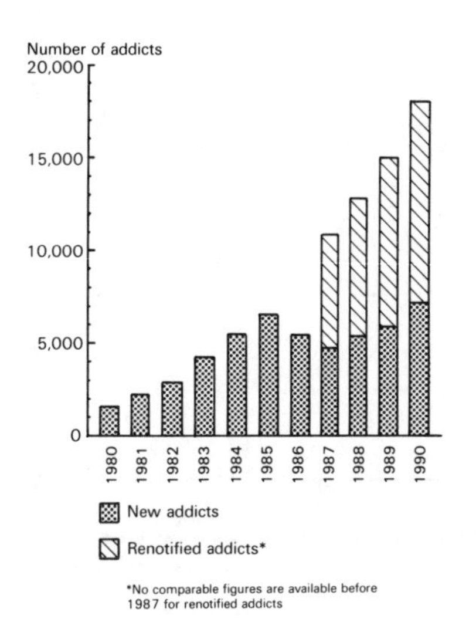

Figure 2.1 Drug addicts notified to the Home Office. United Kingdom, 1980–90.

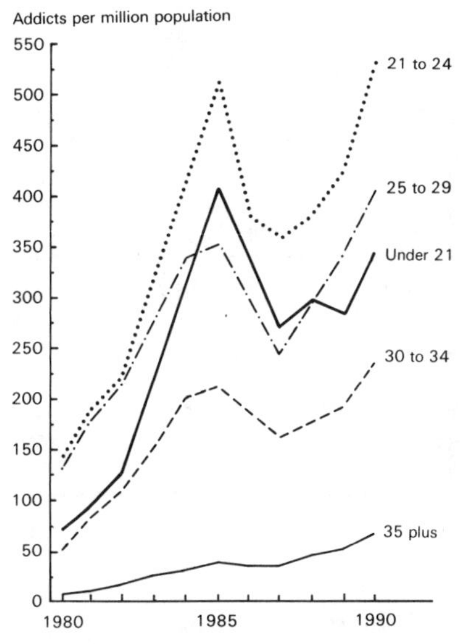

Figure 2.2 New addicts per million population by age, 1980–90

2.2 Which drugs are misused?

Since the first edition of the Guidelines in 1984, patterns of drug misuse have changed. Misuse of opioids remains a growing problem but new drugs of misuse have emerged such as Ecstasy (3,4 methylenedioxymethamphetamine, MDMA for short) crack (cocaine) and Temgesic (buprenorphine). Other drugs such as hallucinogens and solvents continue to be misused. Barbiturate misuse previously constituted a major problem but is now rare. The place of the barbiturates has been taken by the benzodiazepines, which have become widely misused, particularly in the form of temazepam by injection.

Table 2.1 Common drugs of misuse

Type of drug	*Examples*	*Risk that the drug will be injected?*	*Drug-specific risks*
opioid	heroin methadone buprenorphine (Temgesic) dipipanone (Diconal)	yes yes yes yes	overdose causes respiratory arrest
sedative/hypnotic	benzodiazepines barbiturates alcohol	yes yes no	fatal overdose withdrawal seizures
stimulant	amphetamines cocaine crack Ecstasy (MDMA)	yes yes no ?yes	disturbed behaviour psychosis
other	cannabis	no	?psychosis

2.3 Who misuses drugs?

Drug misusers are a heterogeneous group. They include:

(i) People, often adolescents, experimenting with drugs or taking them intermittently, who may not be dependent at the time of referral. They may not be aware of any problems, but the risks include:

- HIV or hepatitis B from shared injecting equipment and unsafe sex;
- increasing the frequency of their use and becoming dependent;
- accidental overdose; accidents during intoxication.

(ii) People whose lives are centred on drugs. They are often involved in a drug subculture, and frequently have multiple social and medical problems related to this.

(iii) Stable long-term drug users who have obtained controlled drugs either on prescription for the treatment of their addiction or from illicit sources. They may have maintained considerable stability in their social and working lives, but may present because of legal problems.

(iv) People who initially presented with a psychiatric or medical problem for which drugs were prescribed but who subsequently continue taking the drugs either for the original problem or in order to avoid withdrawal symptoms. The amount of drugs which they consume may be quite stable. They may experience social or legal, as well as physical or psychological, problems.

2.4 What can doctors do?

2.4.1. Prevention

Doctors should seek to ensure that patients understand the dangers of drug misuse and dependence, particularly those patients who are at special risk, for example:

- young people who live in an area with a high prevalence of drug misuse
- patients receiving a new prescription for benzodiazepines.

The doctor's own careful prescribing habits can help reduce the risk that patients will misuse or become dependent on prescribed drugs such as benzodiazepines.[6]

2.4.2 *Responding to a problem of drug misuse*

As with other medical problems, there are straightforward elements of the clinical management of drug misuse which can be taken on by any doctor

eg treatment of intercurrent infection, short to medium term prescribing of oral methadone for opioid addiction.

More complicated interventions are best tackled by doctors with the relevant specialised training, expertise and back-up

eg prescribing of injectable drugs.

3 Principles of Clinical Management
(applicable to all doctors)

The same basic principles of clinical management apply to all forms of drug misuse.

3.1 Why bother?

- Drug misuse is a substantial and growing problem.
- Every doctor is now likely to encounter patients who misuse drugs.
- In a substantial proportion of patients, drug misuse tends to improve with time. Skilled management keeps the patient healthy and encourages the process of recovery.
- Patients who continue to use drugs can be helped to reduce the risk of HIV infection or other harm.

3.2 General considerations

Drug misusers have the same entitlement as other patients to the services provided by the NHS. It is the responsibility of all doctors to provide care for both general health needs and drug-related problems, whether or not the patient is ready to withdraw from drugs. Every doctor must provide medical care to a standard which could reasonably be expected of the average practitioner in his position. This should now be taken to include provision of the more straightforward treatments for drug misuse such as the prescription of oral methadone for patients dependent on opioids.

The management and treatment of drug misusers present medical practitioners with some particular challenges. The medical problems which may arise are influenced by the nature and dose of the drug, the route by which it is taken and the duration of the habit. Intoxication with drugs may mask Underlying physical problems such as a head injury.

Table 3.1 Medical complications of drug misuse

● **hazards of the drug**	overdose psychosis withdrawal seizures	
● **hazards of injecting**	viral infections; HIV1, HIV2, hepatitis B, C and D septicaemia pneumonia pulmonary abcess infective endocarditis skin abcesses	 osteomyelitis thrombophlebitis gangrene allergic reactions

Doctors often have the impression that patients who misuse drugs are difficult and unresponsive to help. In fact, drug misuse is at least as responsive to treatment as familiar medical conditions such as diabetes or rheumatoid arthritis. Outcome studies show that, with effective care, about 30–40% of opioid misusers will become abstinent and many of the others will be using less heavily or less dangerously. In general, a shorter history of drug misuse carries a better prognosis.[7]

3.2.1 Service needs

Some patients will want help in getting off drugs. Some drug misusers may not acknowledge that they have any health or personal problems related to drug use. Some may be unwilling or unable to give up drugs at the present time but need help to reduce the risks associated with continued drug use.

There is a special need to provide services to HIV-positive drug misusers and those who are at high risk of HIV infection. This demands collaboration particularly between general practitioners, drug misuse treatment services, genito-urinary medicine services and infectious disease units. As with all patients, doctors need to take adequate precautions against transmission of HIV or other viral infections during assessment and treatment.[8]

3.2.2 *Clinical management*

implies a broadly-based approach to care in which the doctor tries to deal with the medical problems of the person who is misusing drugs. This may, for example, involve the prescription of antibiotics for an infection or a controlled drug to aid withdrawal. Increasingly, it will involve liaison with other professionals, such as a practice nurse, a community psychiatric nurse, a social worker or a counsellor from a specialist drug agency. The approach needs to strike a balance between maintaining a humane response to people in real need and limiting the risk that the patient will abuse the service.

Patients need to feel confident of a sympathetic hearing and the availability of effective care, but must be helped to understand that a prescription is not always necessary or useful.

Treatment is not the same as prescribing a substitute for the drug of dependence, though this is often part of the process. Where a prescription is offered, it should form part of a comprehensive package of care.

The aim of clinical management is to help the patient to:

- deal with problems related to drug use;
- reduce the damage during drug use, particularly the risk of HIV (eg from injecting and sharing);
- reduce the chance of future relapse to drug use;
- reduce the duration of episodes of current drug use and of relapses;
- remain healthy until, with appropriate care, he can achieve a drug- free life.

3.2.3. *Support services*

including voluntary agencies, family and friends, may have a crucial role to play in helping with problems of accommodation, employment and personal relationships. It is important for the doctor to be aware of what local

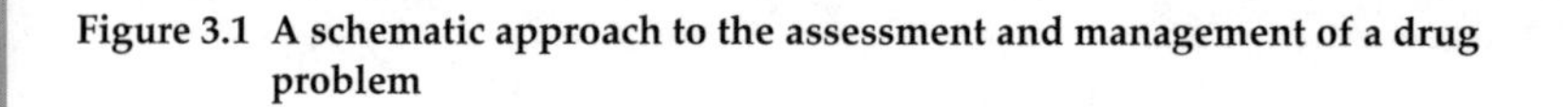

Figure 3.1 A schematic approach to the assessment and management of a drug problem

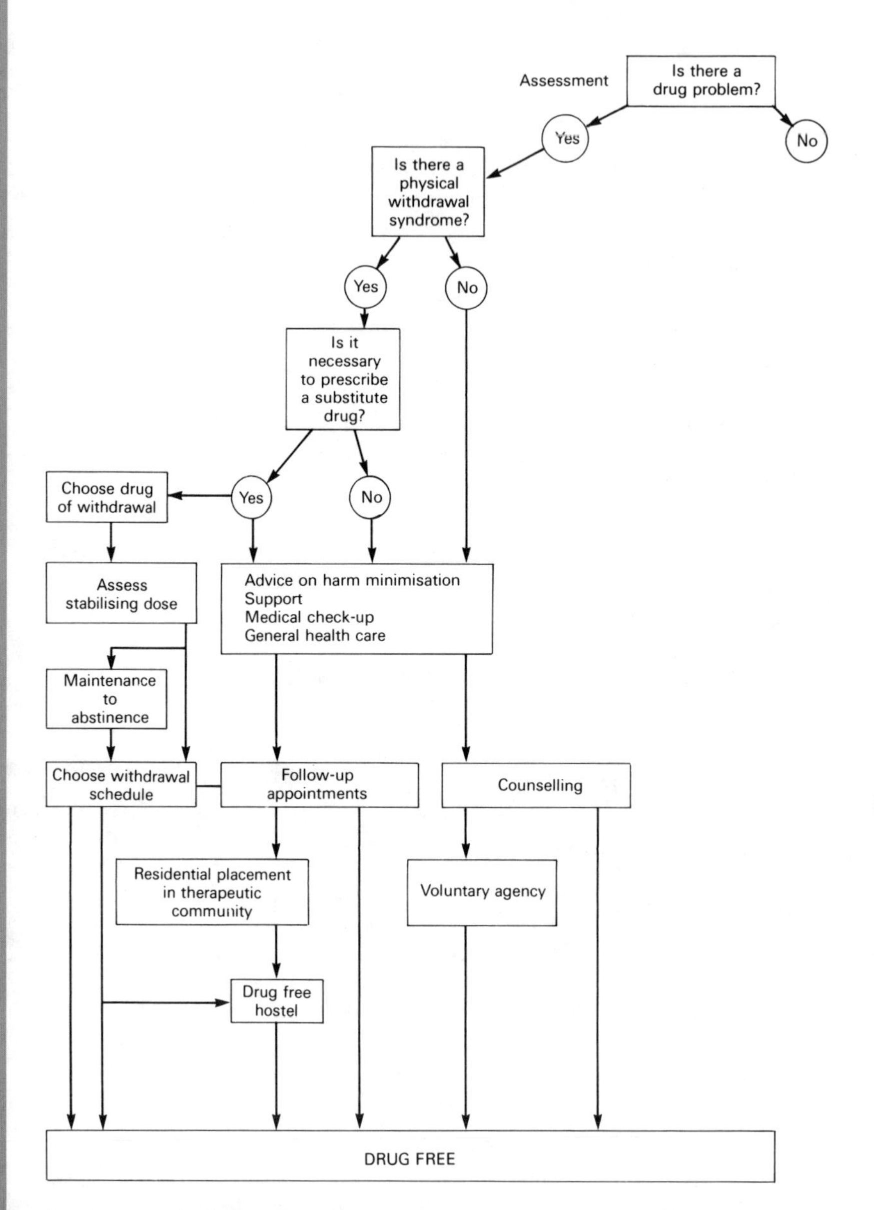

services are available in the statutory, voluntary and private sectors. Local information may be obtained from the Secretary of the District Drug Advisory Committee, from local medical organisations or from a directory of services such as those listed in at the end of this document.

3.2.4 The distinction between assessment and treatment

is made in the interest of clarity. In practice, treatment begins with the first contact and assessment continues throughout. The extent of assessment should be proportional to the nature of the anticipated treatment. Thus the period of assessment for a brief prescription of oral methadone mixture can be shorter than the assessment before undertaking longer-term prescribing.

3.3 Assessment

Drug misusers may be referred to a doctor via many different routes. They may be referred by a social worker, police officer, probation officer or other professional worker in a statutory or voluntary agency. Many patients are self-referred, seeking help for withdrawal symptoms (see Appendix 1), for medical problems, or to get off drugs. Others are referred by relatives or friends, who may accompany the patient to the surgery or hospital. In some cases there may be an impending court case. The outcome for patients referred through the criminal justice system can be just as good as for patients who self-refer.

Most patients who present with a drug problem are serious about needing help. Some drug misusers may present with spurious physical symptoms, eg backache or dysmenorrhoea, hoping to obtain a prescription for the desired drug. Some patients aim to obtain a prescription for more drugs than they themselves require in order to sell the surplus on the black market.

Patients may consult a doctor for a medical problem without mentioning a habit of drug misuse. Doctors should be prepared to enquire about drug use, perhaps as part of a general screening which leads on from questions about other health-related habits such as diet, exercise, drinking, smoking and use of medication. Increased awareness among doctors of the possibility of drug misuse, and a matter-of-fact non-judgemental attitude, will encourage appropriate enquiries and disclosure.

The treatment which a patient asks for may be different from the treatment which the doctor judges to be appropriate. This is particularly true for drug misusers whose addiction may lead them to confuse good care with a ready supply of drugs. The patient's wishes should form the starting point, but not the end point, for the doctor's assessment of what is likely to be helpful.

Table 3.2 Assessing the drug user

In assessing the drug user, ask:

- Type of drug used, quantity, frequency and route?
- Tolerance, dependence and withdrawal?
- Know that sharing transmits HIV?
- What HIV risk?
- Ever use someone else's needle or syringe?
- Ever lent syringe?
- Share with partner only?
- Who does partner share with?
- Source of clean syringes/needles?
- Cleaning technique?
- Could they stop injecting?
- Sites of injecting?
- Any physical problems as a result?
- Sexual activity safe or unsafe?
- Pregnant?
- Ever use a condom?
- Prostitution?

From "Minimising HIV Infection in Drug Users" by M. Farrell and J. Strang

The nature of the first consultation will depend upon whether or not the doctor is aware that the patient is seeking advice about a drug- related problem. If this is known, it may be helpful to offer a longer appointment which allows enough time for a full diagnostic interview and physical examination. Concerned relatives or professionals already involved should be encouraged to attend with the patient.

Often, the patient will attend without forewarning of the problem. In these circumstances the doctor should provide what help he can in the time available and offer a further interview as soon as possible. The doctor should explain to the patient the need for a fuller evaluation of the problem before deciding on appropriate longer-term treatment.

Table 3.3 Features which suggest possible drug misuse

How the patient presents for help	With a specific request for drugs of abuse. Outside normal GP surgery hours. As a temporary resident.
Symptoms and signs	Puncture marks, scars and pigmentation over injection sites. Pupils markedly constricted or dilated. Unexplained constipation or diarrhoea.
Behaviour during consultation	Unaccountably drowsy, elated or restless. Loss of former interest in appearance or work.
Social behaviour	Family disruption. Frequent changes of GP. History of offences to obtain money.

The diagnosis of drug use itself is of central importance. Before treatment is initiated, the doctor should try to check that the history of drug use given by the patient is genuine. Information from other sources, including family, friends and other professionals involved, may be of considerable value. It may be difficult to complete an assessment on the first meeting because frankness on the patient's part depends on the establishment of trust, and may be distorted by perceived secondary gain.

A careful history and physical examination is essential. History-taking should include present and past patterns of drug use, description of situations which precipitate drug use and degree of HIV risk-taking behaviour. Physical examination involves checking for stigmata of drug use (e.g. needle marks) and for evidence of co- morbidity (e.g. Hepatitis B, HIV illness) as well as signs of intoxication, dependence or withdrawal.

At the first interview, advice on harm minimisation (see 3.5.1) and any immediate treatment for medical conditions should be given. Where necessary, arrangements should be made for special investigations e.g. liver function tests, screening for hepatitis B, and screening of urine for drugs. The patient may need access to a supply of injecting equipment or condoms. The doctor may provide these or direct the patient to an appropriate agency. 2 ml syringes and 25 gauge (orange) needles are suitable.

Urine testing is generally more helpful than blood testing because it provides a view of drug use over a longer period of time. It is sensible to request urine testing for a wide range of drugs, including opioids, amphetamines, cocaine, and sedatives such as the benzodiazepines. The screen should not be limited to the drug use claimed by patient. If the doctor suspects that the patient may attempt to falsify the urine sample to give misleading results, the sample should be collected under observation and tested for temperature to verify that it is fresh. Blood tests can be of particular value to measure levels of sedative and hypnotic drugs. A breathalyser will give information on alcohol levels. The smell of solvents on the patient's breath is indicative of their recent inhalation.

Advice on the collection and transport of blood and urine samples should be sought from the local hospital laboratory services. To avoid the risk of infection, adequate precautions should be taken against contamination during venepuncture and leakage from the container during transport. Forms and containers should be appropriately marked with warning labels.

A further aid to assessment is the Home Office Addicts Index (see paragraph 3.4 and Appendix 2) which holds confidential clinical information about addicts. If the patient has previously been notified, the Index can provide the doctor with the names of previous doctors who can then be contacted by the new doctor for information about the past history of drug misuse and treatment. The doctor should let the patient know that he will follow the usual medical procedure of consulting the patient's previous doctor or other doctors currently providing care.

3.4 Notification and Reporting.

3.4.1 Notifying the Addicts Index

The Chief Medical Officer maintains the Addicts Index at the Home Office. The purposes of the Index are to:

- assist doctors in their clinical management of patients
- provide epidemiological data to follow trends in drug misuse
- monitor prescribing for drug misusers
- assist in the planning of services.

All doctors have a statutory obligation to notify the Chief Medical Officer of any contact with a patient known or suspected to be addicted to any of the list of specified opioids or cocaine (see A2.1).

3.4.2 *Reporting to the local Drug Misuse Database*

A system of local Drug Misuse Databases has been established, operated by each Regional Health Authority in England, and by the Common Services Agencies in Wales and in Scotland (see A2.2).

In most parts of the country, completion of a single form allows a doctor to report to the Database and, where appropriate, fulfil the statutory obligation to notify the Chief Medical Officer.

3.4.3 *Confidentiality and informing the patient*

The doctor should inform the patient that anonymised information will be supplied to the local Drug Misuse Database and that there is a legal obligation on the doctor to notify the Chief Medical Officer of patients addicted to some opioids and cocaine. The patient should be reassured that both the Regional Databases and the Addicts Index maintain strict standards of confidentiality and that personal details are not available to the police, for example.

3.5 Treatment

At present, only a minority of drug misusers are in contact with treatment services at any given time. The emergence of HIV infection among injecting misusers and the threat of spread to the community at large has made it even more important than before to attract more drug misusers into treatment.

3.5.1 *Reducing the harm* **("harm minimisation").**

Doctors are familiar with the need to reduce the damage produced by a habit which the patient cannot or will not give up: for example, smokers may be advised to switch to low tar or filter-tips, or to cut down, if they are not ready to stop smoking altogether.

Drug misuse has features in common with hypertension, diabetes and other chronic medical conditions. As with these illnesses, skilful clinical management will reduce the harm to the patient from drug misuse. The term "harm minimisation" has recently been adopted to describe this approach but the underlying principles are a long-established part of good medical practice.

Table 3.4 Aims of harm minimisation

Drug-related goals	Broader goals
• stop or reduce use of contaminated injecting equipment	• stop or reduce unsafe sex
• stop or reduce sharing of injecting equipment	• encourage health consciousness
	• encourage a more stable way of life
• stop or reduce drug misuse	• establish and retain contact

Table 3.5 Harm minimisation strategies.

Education	• hazards of injecting drug misuse (especially sharing injecting equipment) • safer sex • how to obtain sterile injecting equipment and condoms • how to clean injecting equipment if it must be re-used (Fig 3.2) • dangers of overdose • First Aid for drug misusers who become unconscious
Direct Action	• hepatitis B immunisation for non-immune individuals • provision of sterile injecting equipment (preferably in exchange for used injecting equipment) • provision of condoms • offer of HIV testing (with appropriate pre- and post-test counselling) • prescription of substitute oral drugs (3.5.3 and Appendix 1)

The doctor should always look for ways to reduce the harm from continued drug use. This approach is applicable across the range of drug-taking behaviour, including injecting heroin use, oral benzodiazepine use, and inhalation of volatile substances. Those patients who are unwilling or unable at present to achieve stable abstinence can nevertheless reduce the risks to themselves and others. Patients who are already trying to give up drugs need the knowledge and the means to limit damage if lapses occur.

3.5.2 Infectious diseases.

Doctors who will be carrying out surgical procedures or other interventions during which blood-borne viruses might be transmitted should take appropriate precautions to prevent infection (Expert Advisory Group on AIDS 1990). Patients should be informed of the reason for precautions.

HIV:

- doctors should keep abreast of current trends in the management of HIV infection.
- doctors should be aware of the need for health care and immunological monitoring for people who are HIV positive.
- doctors should offer HIV antibody testing and counselling or have arrangements for rapid referral to a service which can provide this.
- early symptoms of HIV disease may mimic drug dependence or withdrawal.

Hepatitis:

- patients should be tested for hepatitis B and C markers to assess immunity, past exposure and current infection.
- hepatitis B is spread by shared injecting equipment and by unprotected sex: it is preventable by immunisation and by avoidance of risk activities. Immunisation should be offered to non-immune individuals. Immunisation against hepatitis B also confers protection against hepatitis D.
- hepatitis C and D are spread by sharing injecting equipment and, probably, by sexual transmission.
- individuals who show evidence of hepatitis C infection or persistent hepatitis B infection should be counselled about the need for continued follow-up and possible treatment to prevent progressive liver damage. They may require referral for this purpose to a specialist who deals with liver disease.

Figure 3.2 How to clean injecting equipment if it must be reused

Cleaning used works		
Draw cold water into the syringe and then flush it out (sterile or cooled boiled water is best) Do this twice	COLDWATER	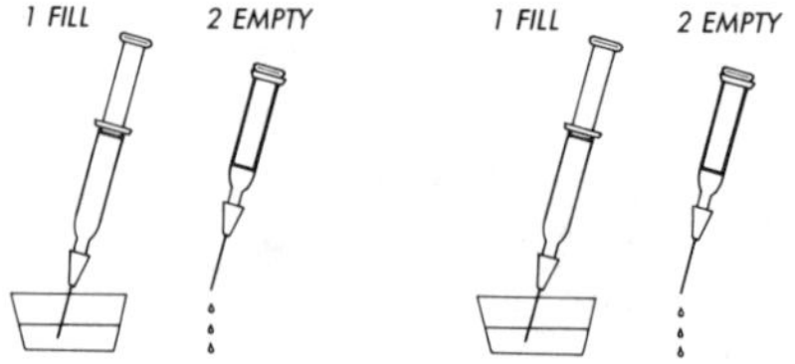 1 FILL 2 EMPTY 1 FILL 2 EMPTY
Draw some household bleach or diluted washing-up liquid into the syringe and flush it out Do this twice as well	BLEACH	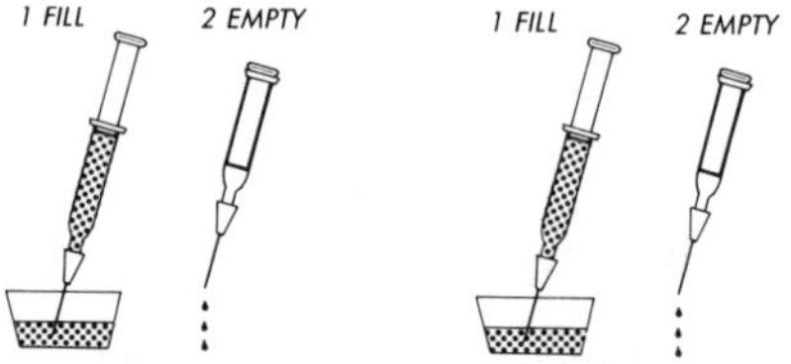 1 FILL 2 EMPTY 1 FILL 2 EMPTY
Finally flush it out twice with fresh water	COLDWATER	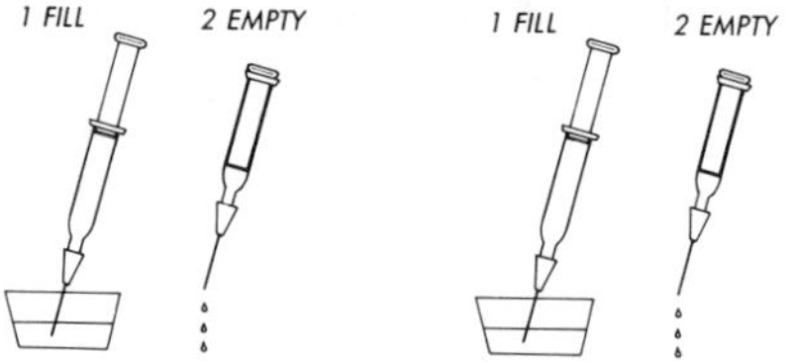 1 FILL 2 EMPTY 1 FILL 2 EMPTY

(adapted from a "Mainliners" leaflet)

3.5.3 *Prescribing*

a. Use of substitute drugs

Drug misuse, even with some degree of dependence, is not in itself an indication to prescribe controlled drugs. Simple reassurance and the prescription of non-controlled drugs may be helpful and effective in alleviating the patient's anxiety about withdrawal (details in Appendix 1).

Prescribing a substitute drug where appropriate can be a useful tool in helping to change the behaviour of some drug misusers either towards abstinence or towards intermediate goals such as a reduction in injecting or sharing of injecting equipment. [9,10]

If opioid drugs are prescribed, liquid oral preparations (eg Methadone Mixture 1mg/ml) are preferable, to avoid the risks associated with injecting crushed tablets or melted suppositories for example, and to reduce the potential for sale on the black market. Some doctors successfully use dihydrocodeine tablets as an alternative to methadone mixture.

Drugs which are capable of injection, such as temazepam capsules, buprenorphine tablets or methadone in tablet form, carry a great risk of being dangerously abused by the patient or sold on the black market. They should not be prescribed to drug misusers.

Any doctor can prescribe methadone and most other opioids to a drug misuser. It is only for the prescription of three specific drugs (cocaine, diamorphine and dipipanone) that a special licence is required (see A2.3)

The most common source of problems in prescribing for drug misusers is the prescription of an open-ended supply of drugs without a clearly agreed goal. Prescribing too little leads to lies and manipulations; too much leads to over-sedation, leakage of surplus drugs to the black market and, in the case of controlled drugs, may bring the doctor to the attention of the Home Office Drugs Inspectorate.

It is important that, when withdrawal is undertaken, it is made clear what the patient will be doing. An agreement or "contract" should be established between the doctor and the patient on the goals they have mutually recognized and when these will be reviewed. For chaotic drug misusers, a month's trial of treatment may be helpful with extension dependent on positive changes.

The doctor should contact a local pharmacist to arrange for the dispensing of a prescription for controlled drugs. Daily dispensing from the pharmacy reduces the risk of overdose or illicit sale of surplus drugs. For some controlled drugs, such as methadone mixture 1mg/ml, it is possible to specify daily dispensing of up to two weeks' supply from a single prescription (see A2.3).

Other doctors who may see the patient should be informed, to avoid double prescribing. The patient should be seen on each occasion by the prescribing doctor or a fully informed colleague. Full and accurate records of all prescriptions must be kept.

b. Patterns of prescribing

The distinction between the following patterns of prescribing is drawn to illustrate the underlying principles, but in practice the categories overlap considerably.

Rapid withdrawal (sometimes called detoxification): This is withdrawal over a short period of a few weeks from an opioid or sedative/hypnotic drug by the use of the same drug or a similar drug in decreasing doses. It can sometimes be assisted by the temporary prescription of other drugs to reduce withdrawal symptoms (see A1.2.1).

Gradual withdrawal: As above, but over the longer period of a few months.

Maintenance to Abstinence (long-term withdrawal): while some patients can achieve abstinence rapidly, others require the support of prescribed drugs for longer than just a few months. Longer-term prescribing should be reviewed at regular intervals and should be part of a broader programme of social and psychological support. It should not be a treatment of first choice. A doctor who feels that a patient is likely to require prescription of an opioid drug for more than a few months should seek advice and support from the local specialist in drug misuse.

Maintenance (stabilisation): The practice of prescribing a substitute drug such as oral methadone for an indefinite period of time with no immediate intention of withdrawal has been suggested as a way of helping a drug dependent patient towards a more stable way of life. There is at least a small proportion of patients for whom this is a helpful approach. It is not described further here as it is a specialised form of treatment best provided by, or in consultation with, a specialist drug misuse service.

3.5.4 Patients who don't seem to be getting better.

If the treatment offered seems not to be succeeding, the doctor should review other possible approaches, in particular the option of shared care with the local specialist in drug misuse. This applies equally to non-prescribing interventions where review should include consideration of whether prescribing might be helpful.

Periods of relapse to drug taking commonly occur on the way to abstinence. They should not be regarded as indicative of failure and can offer the opportunity to learn more about factors which influence drug taking behaviour.

If the patient finds he cannot cope with the agreed withdrawal schedule, there should be a reassessment to judge whether or not a longer period of prescribing is appropriate. The doctor should be aware of the risk that this can lead inadvertently to an overall increase in the amount of drug being taken or can establish a pattern of endless prescribing.

In the event of repeated failures, either because the patient continues to use illicit drugs or because of unreasonable behaviour, the doctor may decide against prescribing further for the patient's drug problem. Continued medical care remains the responsibility of that doctor until further referral or transfer of the patient is arranged.

3.6 Responding to a crisis

The swift administration of a specific antidote to a patient who has overdosed can be life-saving. Doctors who may see patients on an emergency basis must ensure ready access to antidotes for opioids (e.g. naloxone).

The Mental Health Act 1983 or the Mental Health (Scotland) Act 1984 can be used to arrange compulsory admission to hospital of a drug misuser who is suffering from a mental disorder (as defined in the Act) which requires his admission in the interests of his own health or safety or that of other people. Drug misuse alone does not constitute a mental disorder. [11,12,13]

3.7 Specialist advice and referral

From time to time a doctor will encounter a patient who seems to require care more specialised or complicated than the doctor could reasonably be expected to provide himself. This cut-off point will vary, depending on the extent of the doctor's own experience in the management of drug misuse and the availability locally of facilities for advice, further training and shared care. As with many medical conditions, the doctor may find it helpful to apply a system of triage to identify those patients who require and will benefit from more specialised help.

Most Districts now have a local specialist service for drug misusers which usually includes a Consultant Psychiatrist and a Community Drug Team. Any doctor who is concerned about a drug misusing patient should be able to obtain advice from or referral to the drug misuse service. The doctor should be aware that onward referral must be handled sensitively to avoid seeming to the patient like rejection.

Table 3.6

Problems which suggest that specialist advice should be sought:	● dependent on several drugs simultaneously ● history of failed treatment attempts ● co-existing serious physical or mental illness (eg HIV disease) ● violent ● seems to require injectable drugs OR high dose of controlled drugs OR cannot tolerate standard substitute drugs.

3.8 Service delivery

The drive to make services more "user-friendly" must remain consistent with the need to maintain clinical standards. The number of drug misusers managed in any one clinical setting should be limited to a level which allows sufficient time for proper assessment and review, permits a therapeutic environment to be maintained and restricts the opportunities for provocations of relapse, such as drug trading between patients. Appointments should be so arranged as to avoid large numbers of drug misusers congregating.

3.9 Security

Doctors and other staff should take sensible precautions to avoid the risk of theft of items such as drugs, prescription pads and headed notepaper. Additional useful suggestions about improving security are listed in the British National Formulary in the section dealing with Controlled Drugs. If a patient threatens violence, it may be necessary to inform the police of the threat.

4 Special Circumstances

The guidance in the following sections is organised on the basis of the particular setting or speciality in which the doctor works.

4.1 The patient in primary care

It was estimated in 1986 that GPs in England and Wales were seeing between 30,000 and 44,000 new cases annually of opioid drug misuse.[14] Most GPs can now expect to encounter several drug misusers every year.The GP is in a specially favourable position to understand a patient's drug problem in the broader context of his life and to extend support to the patient's family.

The GP needs to strike a balance between making help readily accessible to those in urgent need while maintaining appropriate vigilance to avoid abuse of the service.

The current terms of service for general practitioners include the responsibility to give advice in connection with the misuse of drugs including solvents.

The model of choice for clinical management is shared care with the specialist, as is now common in ante-natal services for example. As with any other patient receiving specialist care, the GP retains overall clinical responsibility for the patient.

Many drug misusers are not registered with a general practitioner, and may seek treatment as temporary or private patients. Some patients may register simultaneously with other doctors, possibly under different names, to ensure a regular supply of drugs. The doctor should encourage the patient to register both as a means of securing access to regular medical care and as a way of tracking the patient through the records system.

4.1.1 *The first contact*

Practice receptionists need to understand that motivation fluctuates; a request for urgent help with a drug problem should be handled with an appropriate degree of priority.

It may be helpful to contact the Family Health Services Authority or Health Board to check if the patient is known to them.

4.1.2 *The consultation*

The GP should offer continuing care. This should include further assessment where necessary, continued counselling of the patient and family, and general medical care. Counselling could be undertaken by a counsellor from the Community Drug Team or Drug Dependency Clinic in co-operation with the doctor.

It is important that partners and other doctors who may see the patient should be clear which doctor is responsible for prescribing any drugs which are required.

A pregnant drug misuser should be managed in close collaboration with obstetric services (see 4.4). The contribution of the GP to supervision in the community is particularly important because drug misusers tend to be poor attenders at ante-natal appointments. Post-natal contraception should be offered.

Figure 4.1

Flow chart illustrating potential responses of a general practice to a patient presenting with a possible drug problem

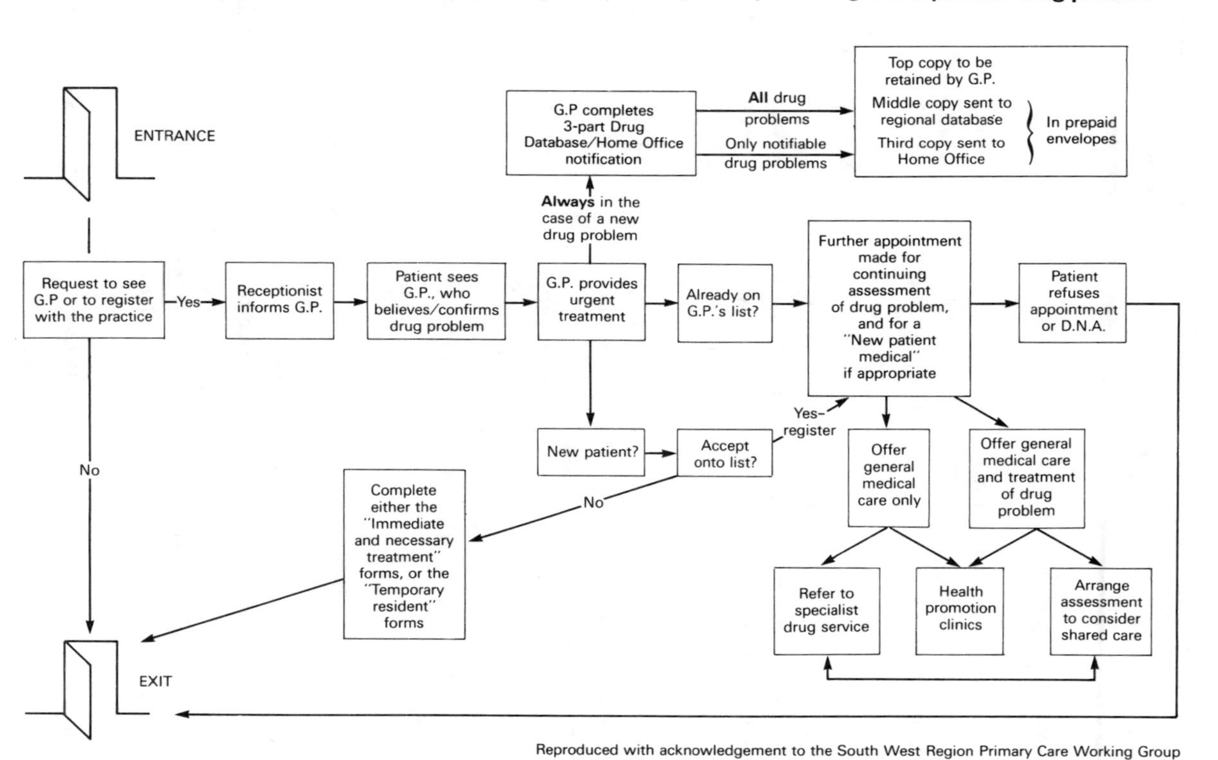

Reproduced with acknowledgement to the South West Region Primary Care Working Group

4.2 Accident and Emergency Care

The A&E medical officer may be the only doctor a drug misuser sees. Many are not registered with a general practitioner and use the A&E department to obtain primary medical care as well as emergency help.

Drug misusers may present to the Accident and Emergency department suffering from acute physical or psychiatric complications of drug misuse. The most immediate concern is likely to be the presenting problem. It is important that investigations (such as urine screens for drugs) are done where possible to help determine the drug status of the patient.

Each A&E department should have a policy on responding to requests from drug misusers for drugs or injecting equipment. The A&E medical officer should prescribe controlled drugs to a drug misuser only where there is a clear medical indication eg the emergency treatment of sedative/hypnotic drug withdrawal or relief of severe physical pain.

A patient brought to hospital following an overdose or whose condition has been sufficiently disturbed to require sedation should be admitted. Early discharge following apparent recovery can be dangerous. It is particularly important to keep a patient under observation if his conscious level has responded to an intravenous injection of naloxone or a benzodiazepine antagonist. These antidotes have shorter half-lives than those of the drugs against which they are administered and there is a risk of the patient relapsing into coma.

Admission to hospital for treatment of medical complications and withdrawal from the drug of dependence is often the most appropriate response. If the patient is not willing to be admitted, the Accident and Emergency medical officer should give treatment for medical conditions and offer referral to other appropriate services. It may occasionally be appropriate to detain the patient under the provisions of the Mental Health Act if there is a co-existing mental disorder (see 3.6).

General psychiatric or specialist drug treatment services should be contacted to advise on the need for urgent referral, and to arrange for a full assessment.

The A&E medical officer should inform the GP of the contact and any treatment or referral, subject to the patient's agreement.

4.3 General Hospital Care

Health problems may require a drug misuser to be admitted to a general medical or surgical ward. The problem may or may not be related to the patient's drug use.

The patient may conceal a drug problem or be too ill to give a clear history. The onset of withdrawal symptoms, particularly in an Intensive Care Unit, can cause diagnostic difficulties.

A drug misuser who is refused necessary medication is likely to discharge himself prematurely or smuggle an independent supply of drugs into hospital. Interaction with prescribed drugs can cause serious interactions or fatal overdose.

Some drug misusers admitted to general hospitals are given the full dose of the drug they claim to need. If the claim is an exaggerated one, the unnecessarily large dose may create a greater degree of dependence on the drug. The correct dose should be calculated by titration against symptoms and signs of withdrawal (see Appendix 1 A1.2.2. and A1.3.1.)

Acutely ill opioid misusers who require analgesics for the relief of organic pain often need larger doses because of their high tolerance to opioid drugs. Previous opioid misuse may be an indication for a more gradual reduction in dose, than in an otherwise comparable patient.

The doctor should consider at an early stage the need for specialist help from the local drug misuse service.

4.4 Pregnancy and Neonatal Care

Obstetricians will increasingly find that they are managing pregnant women dependent on opioids and other drugs. For some women, contact with obstetric services during pregnancy may be their only contact with health services of any kind. The doctor should take this chance to promote harm minimisation. A woman who plans to continue the pregnancy may be more highly motivated at this time to tackle her drug problem.

Each obstetric department should develop a protocol for care of pregnant drug misusers in conjunction with the local drug misuse service and social services.

If a sufficiently high standard of care is attained, no additional infection control measures are needed for the clinical care of women who are known to be HIV positive. However, until this is achieved, some additional precautions will be necessary during care of those women who are known to be HIV positive or who are continuing with high risk behaviour, such as injecting drug misuse.[15]

4.4.1 Ante-natal care

A pregnant woman who misuses drugs has a high risk of obstetric complications. Dates are often uncertain and there is a raised incidence of intrauterine growth retardation and premature labour. Careful clinical supervision is required for both mother and foetus.

The woman should be seen throughout the ante-natal period by the same group of professionals, including a representative from the local drug specialist services.

Drug misusers are often poor attenders. Good liaison between obstetric and drug misuse services and a tolerant, understanding approach increase the chances of retaining contact.

Ante-natal attendance provides an opportunity to offer cervical cytology to women who are likely to be at high risk of cervical intra-epithelial neoplasia but unlikely to have regular cervical smears.

A meeting should be held to plan care. The patient should be informed of this and the reason for it. A woman who feels unable to discontinue drug use is likely to be anxious that her baby may be taken into local authority care. She will benefit from reassurance that drug misuse of itself is not sufficient reason to separate mother and child.[16,17]

The paediatrician should be involved in identifying problems likely to be encountered with the baby and in deciding on the necessary management.

Pregnant women who are HIV positive require specialist counselling on the risks to mother and foetus. Doctors should take appropriate precautions (Expert Advisory Group on AIDS 1990) and should avoid foetal invasive procedures.

Management of the drug problem itself is best done in close liaison with the Drug Dependence Unit. Drug withdrawal is least stressful for mother and foetus if it is done slowly during the mid trimester. If abstinence can be achieved by 4-6 weeks before the birth there is little chance of neonatal withdrawal symptoms. Sudden withdrawal is best avoided because of the risk of intra-uterine death.

4.4.2 Delivery

Appropriate measures should be taken to protect attendants from transmission of blood-borne viruses.[18]

If the patient is receiving a prescription for opioids, these can be continued in labour to provide analgesia. There is no specific contra-indication to the use of epidural anaesthesia. Arrangements should be made to ensure that skilled paediatric care is readily available (see para 4.4.3).

4.4.3 Neonatal paediatric care

The baby of a drug misuser may need skilled paediatric care. This depends on the level of drug use by the mother prior to delivery. Withdrawal symptoms may appear up to a week after delivery and all babies need to be observed during that time. In babies born with a high degree of dependence on opioids, irritability may persist for some weeks and convulsions are possible.

Babies born to HIV positive mothers will need to be followed up to assess their HIV status and the need for treatment.

4.4.4 Postnatal care

Breast feeding is best avoided if the woman is HIV positive, and requires careful consideration if the woman is at high risk of becoming HIV positive or is receiving large doses of opioids.

A meeting should be held soon after delivery to decide the degree of social supervision which will be required when the baby leaves the hospital and the appropriate support for the mother from, for example, the community nurse, midwife or health visitor.

Continuing support is essential after discharge from hospital. Follow- up should involve the general practitioner and also social services in those cases where there is concern for the safety of the child or the mother. There have been reports of a raised incidence of sudden infant death syndrome.

Post-natal contraception should be arranged or offered.

4.5 General Psychiatric Care

4.5.1 General considerations

If there is no local specialist doctor responsible for drug misuse services, a general psychiatrist should act as a source of advice and support for general practitioners and other medical colleagues, and should have knowledge of what treatment resources are available.

Drug misusers may be managed as out-patients, day-patients or in-patients, often in close collaboration with the general practitioner. It is necessary to establish clear agreement as to whether any controlled drugs will be prescribed, and, if so, who will be responsible for prescribing and what regime will be followed.

4.5.2 Drug misuse as co-pathology with mental illness.

In some patients, drug misuse and mental illness co-exist. Acute psychiatric disturbance is an adverse effect of certain drugs (eg psychosis due to LSD or amphetamine). withdrawal from some drugs may lead to affective disturbance (eg anxiety or depression uncovered by discontinuation of benzodiazepines or following withdrawal from stimulants or hallucinogens). Drug misusers with HIV disease may develop neuropsychiatric problems. In other cases, cause and effect is in the opposite direction; drug misuse may follow psychiatric disturbance, perhaps as an attempt to cope with the symptoms of mental illness. It is important to determine which is the primary pathology in order to identify the right treatment. It may be appropriate to transfer some patients to a psychiatrist specialising in drug misuse once the diagnosis is clear.

4.5.3 Drug misuse as presenting problem

In some areas, specialist psychiatrists working in a drug misuse service provide most of the specialist care for drug misusers. Elsewhere, general psychiatrists may provide the bulk of the service. In most Districts and Health Boards there should now be at least one psychiatrist who takes special responsibility for drug misuse services and is able to offer advice and consultation to colleagues.

4.5.4 Admission to a psychiatric unit

This should form part of a planned strategy of clinical management.

It will sometimes be necessary to arrange rapid assessment and urgent admission for a drug misuser. Some patients cannot tolerate withdrawal in the community; others may require stabilisation of a drug regime or treatment of psychiatric illness. There should be provision for mothers and babies.

It is wise to carry out a drug screen as soon as possible after presentation, particularly in the in-patient setting.

Clear operational policies reduce the risk of illicit drug use on the ward and help to avoid disruptive behaviour and management problems. It may be necessary to limit the number of drug misusers admitted at any one time, to restrict or screen visitors, or to require urine testing as part of a treatment contract.

There should be a clear policy on follow up after both planned and unplanned discharge and the conditions under which discharged patients can be re-admitted.

4.5.5 Continuing care

Many patients who misuse drugs require long-term supervision. Continuing care is likely to require collaboration with other agencies such as general practitioners, social workers, probation officers and voluntary organisations. The general psychiatrist may need to act as a co-ordinator to ensure effective inter-disciplinary working.

Some drug misusers benefit from residential placement in a specialist rehabilitation house. The psychiatrist should develop a knowledge of what is available locally and establish good working relationships with the relevant agencies.

Currently, few general psychiatrists receive specific training in the treatment of drug misuse. The Royal College of Psychiatrists has recommended that senior registrar training in substance misuse should be developed in every Region.

4.6 Genito-urinary Medicine (GUM) and HIV Services

Injecting drug misuse is a high-risk behaviour for HIV and hepatitis B infection. Drug misusers may be more likely to engage in unsafe sex while intoxicated or to finance a drug habit.

A drug misuser may present to a GUM physician because of concern over HIV or a sexually-transmitted disease, perhaps with a request for HIV testing. The patient may or may not volunteer a history of drug use.

An HIV positive drug misuser who becomes ill with HIV disease will require help both with HIV-related problems and with drug-related problems. The GUM physician and local doctors who are providing treatment for drug misusers need to have a good working relationship so that each can seek the advice of the other over patients who need both their help. It is important to clarify which doctor is responsible for any prescribing of controlled drugs.

4.7 The Independent Sector

Doctors working in the independent sector should ensure that they have appropriate access to consultation with local NHS colleagues. Doctors in isolated posts should seek peer support from senior medical colleagues in order to maintain consistent standards of good prescribing practice.

Policies on such matters as confidentiality, prescribing and patients with child care responsibilities should be consistent with local NHS and Social Services practice.

Doctors should limit their practice to patients who live within easy reach. It is difficult to maintain good clinical management of patients who live at a great distance from the service.

Doctors should be aware of the potential pitfalls of receiving payment for treatment of drug misuse. A private prescription for controlled drugs may be misconstrued by the patient and others as a supply of drug in exchange for cash. The doctor should seek evidence of patients' ability to pay, by legitimate means, any prescription charges or fees.

The prescription of controlled drugs is best limited to oral methadone mixture or dihydrocodeine. There is a risk that patients may try to finance their consultation and prescriptions by selling higher-value controlled drugs on the black market (see A1.2.2).

4.8 Police Custody

Many drug misusers come into conflict with the law either because of offences committed to finance a drug habit or because of offences under the Misuse of Drugs Act 1971.

A drug misuser who has been detained should be seen as soon as possible by a doctor for assessment. Medical assessment should include whether the patient is fit to be detained or interviewed.

Prompt treatment to limit or prevent withdrawal symptoms will help to reduce the risk of disturbed behaviour in custody and ensure that the patient is fit to be interviewed.

A police surgeon is usually prepared to provide a short-term prescription to allow a sick person in custody to continue the medical treatment which he has been receiving. The same consideration should apply to drug misusers who are receiving a prescription of methadone or another drug as a treatment for drug misuse.

If it seems likely that the patient is dependent on opioids, benzodiazepines or other drugs which produce withdrawal symptoms, then the doctor should prescribe the appropriate treatment to reduce the risk of seizures and the severity of other withdrawal symptoms (see Appendix 1).

Police surgeons have a responsibility to alert police officers with whom they work to:

- the need for adequate observation and supervision
- the early signs of acute withdrawal from opioids, sedative/hypnotic drugs and alcohol
- the dangers of overdose in custody
- the effects of combinations of drugs and alcohol
- emergency resuscitation measures
- appropriate precautions to avoid infection with blood-borne viruses such as HIV and hepatitis.

4.9 Prison

Drug misusers in prison have the same rights as other prisoners to a satisfactory standard of medical and psychiatric care.

4.9.1 Reception to prison

A prisoner may be reluctant to disclose the fact that he is misusing drugs. The doctor should check that the medical questionnaire has been completed on reception and should carry out a medical examination.This will increase the likelihood of disclosure and detection of drug use.

If the history and examination indicate that the prisoner is dependent on drugs, then the doctor should offer a detoxification programme unless there is some specific contra-indication to this. Examples of routine detoxification programmes suitable for use in prison are specified in "Caring for Drug Users."[19]

It may be helpful to seek information from the patient's previous doctor.

4.9.2 Care during prison sentence

The prison doctor should:

- be familiar with relevant local guidance on care of drug misusers
- be a member of any drug throughcare management team.
- ensure that drug misusers receive essential information on harm minimisation (see 3.5.1, Figure 3.2 and Tables 3.4 and 3.5) and on what help is available in prison for drug problems.
- be aware of outside agencies which offer help to drug misusers and refer prisoners to these as appropriate.
- see the prisoner shortly before discharge from prison.
- give appropriate advice on reducing the risks of drug misuse once back in the community, especially the danger of accidental overdose arising from loss of tolerance during enforced abstinence in custody.
- provide a contact in the community for help with drug problems.
- make arrangements for continuity of medical care on the prisoner's return to the community and, where appropriate, refer him to a specialist drug agency.

Some of this information may conveniently be included in a Drug Advisory Card given to the prisoner on discharge.

Appendix 1: Managing Withdrawal

A1.1 General Principles

Withdrawal syndromes differ according to the particular drugs involved, the daily amounts taken, the duration of use and individual sensitivity.

Table A1.1 Two common withdrawal syndromes

Opioids	Benzodiazepines
nausea, vomiting, diarrhoea restlessness, anxiety irritability, sleeplessness	*anxiety symptoms* eg anxiety, sweating, insomnia, headache, shaking, nausea
pains in muscles, bones, joints running nose and eyes, sneezing yawning, sweating	*disordered perception* eg feelings of unreality abnormal body sensations abnormal sensation of movement hypersensitivity to stimuli
dilated pupils, gooseflesh flushing	*major incidents:* psychosis epileptiform seizures

A1.1.1 Psychological support is important

The doctor should help the patient to weigh the benefits of choosing the best time for withdrawal against the risks of continued drug use. If possible, a time of relative stability in the patient's life increases the chance of success. It is useful to have support from family members and/or a therapist. The doctor should involve those close to the patient in the management of the drug problem and help them clarify their responsibilities for supporting the patient.

The severity and management of withdrawal symptoms is greatly influenced by psychological factors present in the treatment setting. Drug withdrawal regimes work best when doctor and patient have got to know each other, and a basic contract about the regime has been mutually agreed. In general, it is best to respond to a patient's own determination and timescale to withdraw from drugs. It may help to reinforce motivation if the doctor can support, as far as it is safe to do so, a patient's wish to come off drugs quickly. If the patient subsequently finds rapid withdrawal too stressful, the doctor can adjust the regime to be more gradual.

At an early stage, doctor and patient should start thinking ahead to longer-term management.

Further psychological support can be provided from voluntary groups. Specific psychological therapy such as cognitive therapy may be of value. It is most likely to be available from specialist mental health services such as community psychiatric nurses and clinical psychologists.

A1.2 Withdrawal from Opioids

A1.2.1 The use of less addictive medication for symptomatic relief

Some patients can be detoxified without substitution of the drug of addiction or a specific withdrawal regime. The use of less addictive drugs for symptomatic relief may be valuable, but should only be used to enhance the psychological support offered by the doctor or others involved. They may also be helpful as an adjunct to a substitution withdrawal programme, where withdrawal symptoms are very severe. The following drugs have been found to be of particular benefit. (Details of prescribing are in the British National Formulary).

Promethazine

An antihistamine with antiemetic and sedative actions. Useful for symptomatic treatment of mild physical withdrawal.

Propranolol

Helpful for patients with pronounced somatic anxiety symptoms. Doses as recommended for general anxiety.

Diphenoxylate and atropine (Lomotil)

Diphenoxylate is a mild opioid with low addictive potential used in the symptomatic treatment of diarrhoea. It may be used to effect with a small dose of thioridazine.

Thioridazine

A phenothiazine tranquilliser with virtually no addictive potential. May be used in low doses to control anxiety. It should not be prescribed for more than two weeks.

Benzodiazepines

These drugs have their own addictive potential. A short course lasting only a few days may help to provide relief from anxiety and insomnia. Prescription should not extend beyond 14 days. Longer-acting forms, eg diazepam, are usually preferable.

A1.2.2 Use of substitute opioids

The substitute drug of choice for opioid misuse is oral Methadone Mixture 1mg/ml. This is effective, long-acting, very unlikely to be injected and has a low resale value on the black market. Dihydrocodeine tablets are sometimes used as an alternative; these have a shorter duration of action and so need to be taken several times a day. There have been reports that dihydrocodeine tablets may be crushed and injected; dihydrocodeine elixir 2mg/ml. is available as an alternative. If the patient cannot tolerate methadone or dihydrocodeine, a referral may be arranged to a specialist drug service, where the validity of his statement may be explored.

Establishing an initial daily dosage

The aim is to find the minimum daily dose that keeps the patient free from withdrawal symptoms. Calculation of the baseline dose can usually be made as an outpatient or in general practice, but may sometimes require a short hospital admission.

It is not possible to convert directly the effects, time duration and addictive potential of opioid-based drugs to a fixed equivalent of methadone. The following table is a rough guide only.

A drug history of the preceding week's drug use, and the use of the opioid/methadone equivalents shown in Table A1.2, will give a reasonable estimate of the initial daily dose of oral methadone.

Table A1.2

Drug	Dose	Methadone equivalent
Street Heroin	Cannot accurately be estimated because street drugs vary in purity. Titrate dose against withdrawal symptoms.	
Pharmaceutical Heroin	10mg tablet or ampoule 30mg ampoule	20mg 50mg
Methadone	10mg ampoule Mixture (1mg/1ml) 10ml Linctus (2mg/5ml) 10ml	10mg 10mg 4mg
Morphine	10mg ampoule	10mg
Dipipanone (Diconal)	10mg tablet	4mg
Dihydrocodeine (DF118)	30mg tablet	3mg
Dextromoramide (Palfium)	5mg tablet 10mg tablet	5-10mg 10-20mg
Pethidine	50mg tablet 50mg ampoule	5mg 5mg
Buprenorphine hydrochloride (Temgesic)	200 microgram tablet 300 microgram ampoule	5mg 8mg
Pentazocine (Fortral)	50mg capsule 25mg tablet	4mg 2mg
Codeine linctus 100ml	300mg codeine phosphate	10mg
Codeine phosphate	15mg tablet 30mg tablet 60 mg tablet	1mg 2mg 3mg
Gee's linctus 100ml	16mg anhydrous morphine	10mg
J.Collis Brown 100ml	10mg extract of opium	10mg

The dose of methadone is then titrated against observable signs of withdrawal eg tachycardia, mydriasis, perspiration and subjective sensations of discomfort. Observable signs should be given greater weight than symptoms.

After 72 hours, the total methadone dose can be summated and divided to calculate a reasonable baseline daily or twice daily dose. This dose can then be used as a starting dose for an inpatient or outpatient detoxification.

Reducing the dose

Steady withdrawal of the drug can be achieved by small daily reductions from the starting dose. A regular stepped reduction in dose is easiest to calculate, though it is probably the rate of reduction which is important. In practice, a more rapid reduction during the early stages and a slower reduction later is often helpful (see Figure Al.l). Most patients will require between 20 and 60 mg of methadone daily. An apparent requirement for a larger dose may indicate the need for advice from a specialist in drug misuse.

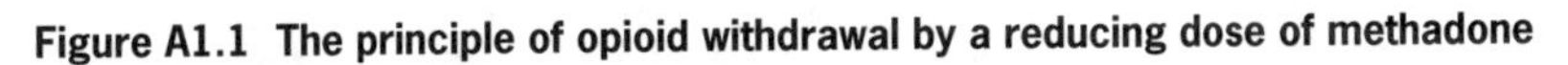

Figure A1.1 The principle of opioid withdrawal by a reducing dose of methadone

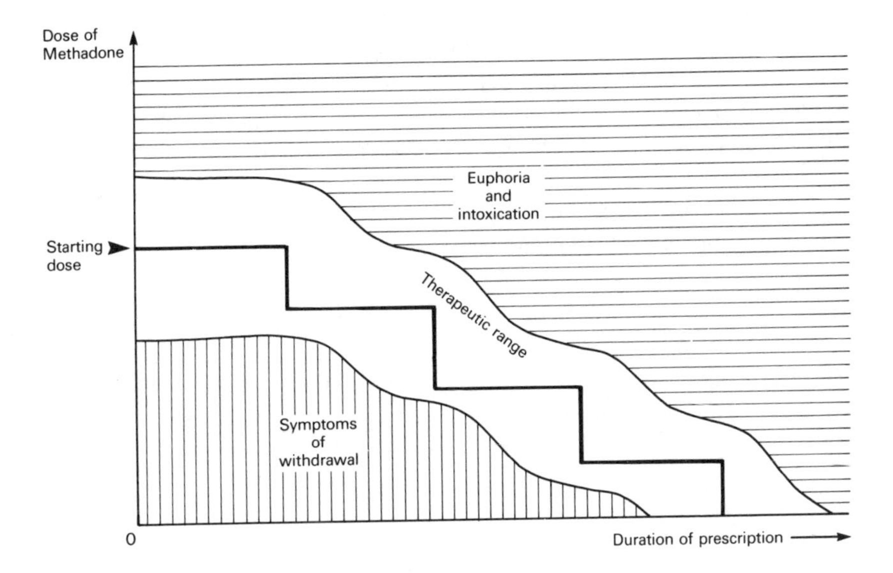

A1.3 Withdrawal from Sedative/Hypnotic Drugs

The following section applies to benzodiazepines and other sedative/hypnotic drugs such as barbiturates and chlormethiazole. Further advice is contained in the British National Formulary. Some patients will be misusing illicitly-obtained drugs; others will have become dependent on prescribed drugs.

A1.3.1 Establishing an initial daily dose

Initially the patient's prescription should be regularised so that daily variations are kept to the minimum. The drug is then reduced steadily until persistent withdrawal symptoms are shown. The dose just above that at which withdrawal symptoms appear is the minimum effective dose. In general it is easier to avoid withdrawal symptoms if a drug is taken only once or twice daily.

A1.3.2 Consider changing to diazepam

Diazepam has a relatively long half-life and is available in many strengths of tablet and as an oral solution. This gives it a number of advantages over other benzodiazepines; it may be given as a once daily dose, is less likely to allow withdrawal symptoms to emerge and readily permits a smooth reduction in dose by small steps. It may be preferable to change to diazepam from the patient's current benzodiazepine over a two-week period. Equivalent doses of common benzodiazepines are indicated in Table A1.3.

A1.3.3 Decide on rate of reduction

Rapid withdrawal

This takes between two and ten weeks and requires close supervision. This usually means in-patient admission or day patient care unless the starting dose is less than 30 mg diazepam or equivalent (see table A1.3.)

Slower withdrawal

This may be spread over several months, perhaps as long as a year. A reduction in dose of around 10% every two weeks is often suitable.

A1.3.4 Is additional medication required?

Additional drugs should be considered only when gradual withdrawal with adequate psychological support has failed. Additional drugs should be prescribed only for a short period as part of a rapid withdrawal programme in order to avoid encouraging long-term use of additional medication. Drugs which may be helpful are:

Propranolol

This can be useful where physical symptoms of anxiety are prominent. Discontinue within four weeks of stopping benzodiazepines. Taper off over one week.

Tricyclic antidepressants (e.g. imipramine, dothiepin)

These can be helpful to reduce severity of withdrawal symptoms and to relieve depression. Start one month before withdrawal begins and continue 1-3 months after benzodiazepines have been stopped. Taper off over 2-4 weeks.

No other drugs have been shown to be of significant benefit in withdrawing from benzodiazepines. **It is important to avoid drugs related to benzodiazepines (eg zopiclone, chlormethiazole and glutethimide) as these drugs are likely to be cross-dependent with benzodiazepines and may substitute one type of sedative drug dependence for another.**

Table A1.3 Approximate dosages of common benzodiazepines equivalent to 5mg diazepam

Drug	Dose
Chlordiazepoxide	15mg
Diazepam	5 mg
Loprazolam	500 micrograms
Lorazepam	500 micrograms
Oxazepam	15 mg
Temazepam	10 mg
Nitrazepam	5 mg

A1.4 Withdrawal from Stimulants

Stimulants such as amphetamines, Ecstasy and cocaine can cause psychological dependence but do not produce a major physical withdrawal syndrome. It is generally best for the patient to discontinue the drugs abruptly. There is usually no advantage in gradual withdrawal.

It is undesirable to prescribe substitute stimulant drugs as the risk of them being misused is very high.

Many drug misusers dependent on stimulants experience insomnia and depression when they stop using the drugs. Antidepressant medication may be required; desipramine has been reported as particularly helpful in these circumstances. Most amphetamine misusers can be managed as outpatients without the use of any medication at all. They will benefit from advice and information on the likely rebound phenomena and the need for a safe place in which to "sleep it off ". Some patients become overtly suicidal and require close observation.

A1.5 Withdrawal from Hallucinogens

Hallucinogenic drugs (e.g. LSD) do not cause physical dependence. It is best to discontinue them abruptly. There is no advantage in gradual withdrawal. It is not necessary to prescribe substitute drugs to allow withdrawal. Symptomatic treatment for psychological symptoms may be of value (e.g. a short course of benzodiazepines to reduce anxiety). Some people who misuse hallucinogens experience severe mental disturbance (see 4.5.2).

A1.6 Withdrawal from Volatile Substances

Volatile substances can be misused by inhalation or sniffing of the vapours to produce a state of intoxication. Substances commonly misused include:

- butane gas (lighter fuel, aerosols)
- solvents (toluene, dry cleaning fluid, typewriter correction fluid)
- glues
- fire extinguisher contents.

There is no physical withdrawal syndrome. It is best to discontinue them abruptly. There is no advantage in gradual withdrawal and no indication to prescribe substitute drugs.

Volatile substance abusers tend to be younger than other types of drug misuser, often school-age children. Many children try sniffing once or twice, but only a small proportion persist and develop a habit. The greatest risk is of sudden death during an episode of sniffing. Butane is particularly dangerous if squirted directly into the mouth as it can cause cardiac arrest. A plastic bag over the face may cause asphyxia. Acute intoxication can lead to fatal accidents through falling or drowning because sniffing is often done out of doors in deserted areas such as stairways or canal banks.

As with other drug misusers, there may well be underlying personal or relationship problems which need to be explored.

The appropriate services for specialist referral and advice are likely to be social services or the local child psychiatrist rather than a drug misuse service. The voluntary agency Re-Solv publishes a national directory of services for people who abuse volatile substances.

A1.7 Withdrawal from Alcohol

Many drug misusers also abuse alcohol and vice versa. Alcohol is a sedative drug and produces a physical withdrawal syndrome. A short course of benzodiazepines or chlormethiazole may be prescribed to prevent the emergence of withdrawal symptoms. Doctors should be aware of the addictive potential of these drugs and of the danger that they may be abused together with alcohol. Further details are given in the British National Formulary and in the publications listed in the reference section under "Alcohol".

A1.8 Cannabis

There are legitimate concerns about the use of cannabis both because it is illegal and because of possible health and safety risks. Misuse of cannabis is not specifically addressed in these Guidelines although many of the same basic principles outlined in Section 3 would apply.

Appendix 2: Notification, Reporting and Prescribing

A2.1 The Home Office Addicts Index

The Misuse of Drugs (Notification of and Supply to Addicts) Regulations 1973 require any doctor to notify the Chief Medical Officer at the Home Office in writing within 7 days if he attends a patient whom he considers to be, or has reasonable grounds to suspect is, addicted to any of the following controlled drugs:

Table A2.1 Controlled drugs which require notification

cocaine	methadone
dextromoramide (palfium)	morphine
diamorphine (heroin)	opium
dipipanone (a constituent of Diconal)	oxycodone
hydrocodone	pethidine
hydromorphone	phenazocine
levorphanol	piritramide

A person is regarded as being addicted to a drug if he has, as a result of repeated administration, become so dependent upon the drug that he has an overpowering desire for the administration of it to be continued.

The name, address, sex, date of birth and National Health Service Number of the patient (if known), together with the date of attendance and the name of the drug or drugs concerned, must be given. Notification does not imply that a prescription has been or will be given. It is helpful if the doctor states whether or not the patient injects and what drugs have been prescribed.

These notifications are compiled in the Addicts Index, which is used to provide epidemiological data to assist the development of national policies and local services for the management of the drug problem, and to allow a doctor to check whether a notifiable drug user is seeking simultaneous treatment from more than one doctor.

Doctors may make enquiries of the Index by telephone. Information is available only to the doctor actually providing care for the patient, on a call-back system, following checks made by the Home Office Drugs Branch on the authenticity of the enquirer. (Home Office Drugs Branch, 50 Queen Anne's Gate, London SW1H 9AT.) Enquiries can be made during working hours on 071-273 2213. An answering machine will take messages out of hours.

Further information is contained in the British National Formulary.

A2.2 Regional Drug Misuse Databases

The Regional Drug Misuse Databases rely on voluntary reporting by doctors and others of details of contacts with patients who have any type of recent drug problem. The Databases therefore contain information about a wider range of drug misuse than is covered by the Addicts Index (eg benzodiazepines and amphetamines are included). Information on pattern of contacts will be fed back to doctors and other reporting agencies. The value of the information will be to allow more accurate planning of services for drug misusers and to monitor the emergence of new patterns of drug misuse. The system is designed to protect the anonymity of patients and does not allow the identification of individuals.

Forms for reporting to the Regional Database are available from the local Family Health Service Authority or Regional Health Authority in England, from the Common Services Agency in Wales, and from the Health Board or the Information and Statistics Division of the Common Services Agency in Scotland.

A2.3 Prescribing controlled drugs

Misuse of Drugs Regulations 1985 require that prescriptions for controlled drugs listed in schedules 1, 2 or 3 (except phenobarbitone, phenobarbitone sodium, and preparations containing them) must be in ink or otherwise indelible and must be signed by the doctor with his usual signature and dated by him. The patient's name and address, the dose to be taken, the form and, where appropriate, strength of a preparation and the total quantity or, in the case of a preparation, the number of dosage units must be in the doctor's own handwriting. If a prescription is to be dispensed by instalments, the prescription must also specify in the doctor's own handwriting the number of instalments, the quantity per instalment and the intervals to be observed. Further information and a specimen completed prescription are contained in the British National Formulary in the section on Prescribing Controlled Drugs.

Special prescription forms exist to allow daily dispensing from a single prescription of certain controlled drugs such as methadone. Hospital practitioners can use the pink prescription form FP10HP(Ad) (in Scotland HBP(A)) on which 14 days prescription can be written conveniently for daily dispensing (two days supply on Saturdays). In England and Wales, general practitioners can use the blue form FP10 (MDA) for the same purpose. In Scotland, GPs use the form GP10 and indicate the number of daily instalments to be dispensed.

Practitioners who are prescribing for ten or more drug misusers may be granted exemption from the handwriting requirements on application to the Home Office Drugs Branch.

Doctors require a special licence from the Home Secretary to administer, supply, authorise the administration or supply of, or prescribe cocaine, diamorphine or dipipanone to a person addicted to any of the drugs notifiable under the 1973 Regulations. Cocaine, diamorphine and dipipanone include their salts and any preparations or other product containing these drugs or their salts. A licence is not required if the administration of cocaine, diamorphine, or dipipanone to an addict or any other person is for the purpose of treating organic disease or injury.

(More detailed guidance is available in the Guide to the Misuse of Drugs Act 1971 and the Misuse of Drugs Regulations[20])

7. REFERENCES

1. Standing Medical Advisory Committee to the Secretaries of State for Health and for Wales (1989).
Drinking problems: a challenge for every doctor. Stanmore (Middlesex): Department of Health.

2. Scottish Home and Health Department (1985).
Slainte Mhath ("Good Health"). The medical problems of excessive drinking. Edinburgh: SHHD.

3. Edwards G, Arif A, Hodgson R. (1981).
Nomenclature and classification of drug and alcohol-related problems:
a WHO memorandum. *Bulletin of the World Health Organisation*; 59 (2): 225-242.

4. Advisory Council on the Misuse of Drugs (1982).
Treatment and Rehabilitation: report. London: HMSO.

5. Home Office Statistical Bulletin (1990).
Statistics of the misuse of drugs: addicts notified to the Home Office, United Kingdom 1990. *Home Office Statistical Bulletin*, issue 8/91. London: Home Office.

6. Welsh Committee on Drug Misuse (1991).
Benzodiazepines: the problem of misuse and dependence. Cardiff: Welsh Office.

7. Ghodse A. H. (1989).
Drugs and addictive behaviour: a guide to treatment. Oxford: Blackwell Scientific publications.

8. UK Health Departments (1990).
Guidance for health care workers: protection against infection with HIV and hepatitis viruses: recommendations of the Expert Advisory Group on AIDS. London: HMSO.

9. Advisory Council on the Misuse of Drugs (1988).
AIDS and drug misuse: part 1. 47-53. London: HMSO.

10. Strang J. (1990).
Intermediate goals and the process of change, in Strang J., Stimson G.V., eds. *AIDS and drug misuse: the challenge for policy and practice in the 1990s*. London: Routledge.

11. DHSS (1987).
The Mental Health Act 1983: memorandum on parts I-VI, VIII and X. London: HMSO.

12. Department of Health and Welsh Office (1990).
The Mental Health Act 1983 code of practice. London: HMSO.

13. Scottish Home and Health Department (1990).
Mental Health (Scotland) Act 1984: code of practice. Edinburgh: HMSO.

14. Glanz A., Taylor C. (1986).
Findings of a national survey of the role of general practitioners in the treatment of opiate misuse: extent of contact with opiate misusers. *British Medical Journal*; 293: 427-430.

15. Royal College of Obstetricians and Gynaecologists (1990).
HIV infection in maternity care and gynaecology. (Revised report of the RCOG Sub-Committee on problems with AIDS in relation to obstetrics and gynaecology). London: RCOG.

16. Standing Conference on Drug Abuse (SCODA) (1989).
Drug using parents and their children: the second report of the National Local Authority Forum on Drug Misuse in conjunction with the Standing Conference on Drug misuse. London: Association of Metropolitan Authorities.

17. Social Services Inspectorate (1991).
Community based services for people who misuse drugs: a study in North-Western region. London: Department of Health.

18. Brettle R., Farrell M., Strang J. (1990).
Clinical features of HIV infection and AIDS in drug takers, in Strang J., Stimson G.V., eds. *AIDS and drug misuse: the challenge for policy and practice in the 1990s*. London: Routledge.

19. Home Office (1991).
Caring for drug users - a multi-disciplinary resource manual for people working with prisoners. (Not available to the general public). London: Home Office.

20. Department of Health, Welsh Office and Scottish Home and Health Department (1989).
Guide to the Misuse of Drugs Act 1971 and the misuse of drugs regulations. Heywood (Lancashire): Department of Health.

FURTHER READING

Drug misuse and dependence

Advisory Council on the Misuse of Drugs (1984).
Prevention: report. London: HMSO.

Advisory Council on the Misuse of Drugs (1988).
AIDS and drug misuse: part 1. London: HMSO.

Advisory Council on the Misuse of Drugs (1989).
AIDS and drug misuse: part 2. London: HMSO.

Banks A., Waller T.A.N. (1988).
Drug misuse: a practical handbook for GPs. Oxford: Blackwell Scientific publications.

Community Drug Project (CDP) (1988).
Safer drug use: the users' Guide. London: Institute for the Study of Drug Dependence.

Department of Health and the Welsh Office. Institute for the Study of Drug Dependence (1985).
Drug misuse: a basic briefing. (A guide for professionals, parents and others who need to know more about drugs and their effects). Stanmore (Middlesex): DHSS.

Ghodse A.H., Maxwell D., eds. (1990).
Substance abuse and dependence: an introduction for the caring professions. London: Macmillan Press.

Glanz A. (1986).
Findings of a national survey of the role of general practitioners in the treatment of opiate misuse: views of treatment. *British Medical Journal*; 293: 543-545.

Glass I.B., ed. (1991).
The international handbook of addiction behaviour. London: Routledge.

Grantham P. (1987).
Benzodiazepine abuse. *British Journal of Hospital Medicine*; 37: 292-300.

Higgitt A., Lader M., Fonagy P. (1985).
Clinical management of benzodiazepine dependence. *British Medical Journal*; 291: 688-690.

Institute for the Study of Drug Dependence (ISDD) (1990).
Drugs, pregnancy and childcare. (A guide for professionals). London: ISDD.

Livingstone M.G. (1991).
Benzodiazepine dependence: avoidance, detection and management. *Prescribers' Journal*; 31(4): 149-156.

Onyett S.R. (1989).
The benzodiazepine withdrawal syndrome and its management. *Journal of the Royal College of General Practitioners*; 39: 160-163.

Royal College of Psychiatrists (1987).
Drug scenes: a report on drugs and drug dependence. London: RCPsych.

Royal College of Psychiatrists (1989a).
Report on services and training from the Executive Committee of the Substance Misuse Section. *Bulletin of the Royal College of Psychiatrists*; 13: 150.

Royal College of Psychiatrists (1989b).
District level services for drug takers. *Bulletin of the Royal College of Psychiatrists*; 13: 322-325.

Strang J., Farrell M. (1991).
Drugs work: hepatitis.. London: Institute for the Study of Drug Dependence.

Strang, J., Stimson G.V., eds. (1990).
AIDS and drug misuse: the challenge for policy and practice in the 1990s. London: Routledge.

Alcohol Misuse

Alcohol Concern and Health Education Authority (1987).
Cut down on your drinking. (Pack containing booklets for doctors to hand out to patients, surgery poster and handbook for health professionals). London: HEA.

Medical Council on Alcoholism (1987).
Hazardous drinking: a handbook for general practitioners. London: Medical Council on Alcoholism.

Health Education Board for Scotland (1990).
DRAMS Scheme: helping problem drinking – resources for general practitioners. Edinburgh: Health Education Board for Scotland.

VIDEO LEARNING PACKS

Health Departments of Great Britain and NHS Training Authority (1985).
Working with Drug Users. A video training package for professionals. 3 hours of video plus associated printed material. Video available for purchase or free loan from the library of the Central Office of Information, Hercules Road, London SE1 7DU. Tel: 071-928 2345

BMA Foundation for AIDS, in association with the Wellcome Foundation (1990).
HIV and Drug Misuse. Booklet and accompanying 15-minute video are available from BMA for purchase or hire. General Practitioners may arrange a free showing of the video by contacting the Wellcome Foundation Marketing Services Manager on 0270 583151.

DIRECTORIES OF SERVICES FOR DRUG MISUSERS

Scotland

Scottish Health Education Group and Scottish Drugs Forum (1991).
Drug problems: a register of helping agencies 6th edition. Edinburgh: Scottish Health Education Group.
Available from: The Health Education Board for Scotland, Woodburn House, Canaan Lane, Edinburgh EH10 4SG.
Tel: 031-447 8044.

England and Wales

Details of local services available on enquiry from:
Standing Conference on Drug Abuse (SCODA),
1-4 Hatton Place, London EC1N 8ND.
Tel: 071-430 2341/2

Services for volatile substance misusers

Re-Solv (1991).
Solvent and volatile substance abuse 2nd edition.
Stone (Staffs.): Re-Solv: the society for the prevention of solvent and volatile substance abuse.
The Re-Solv National Directory available from: The Society for the Prevention of Solvent and Volatile Substance Abuse, St Mary's Chambers, 19 Station Rd, Stone, Staffordshire ST15 8JP.
Tel: 0785-817885.

OTHER USEFUL ADDRESSES

Institute for the Study of Drug Dependence (ISDD), 1 Hatton Place, London EC1N 8ND.
Tel: 071-430 1991.
Provides a reference library and information service free to anyone with an interest in the topic of drug misuse. Produces useful, up-to-date leaflets and publications on a wide range of drugs and related subjects.

Scottish Drugs Forum, 5 Oswald St., Glasgow G1 4QR.
Tel: 041-221 1175.

Printed in the United Kingdom for HMSO.
Dd.0295153, 12/91, C1000, 3385/4, 5673, 173792.